Table of Contents

I. Introduction
   A. Definition and history of essential oils
   B. Discuss the growing interest in natural wellness and alternative therapies
   C. State the purpose of the book and what readers can expect

II. Understanding Essential Oils
   A. What are essential oils and how are they extracted?
   B. The science behind essential oils and their chemical composition
   C. Different types of essential oils and their properties
   D. Safety precautions and guidelines for using essential oils

III. Exploring the Benefits of Essential Oils
   A. Physical Benefits
      1. Supporting the immune system and overall wellness
      2. Relieving pain and inflammation
      3. Promoting relaxation, stress reduction, and better sleep
      4. Supporting healthy digestion and detoxification
      5. Enhancing skin health and beauty

   B. Emotional and Mental Benefits
      1. Uplifting mood and reducing anxiety, stress, and depression
      2. Enhancing focus, concentration, and mental clarity
      3. Supporting emotional balance and well-being
      4. Boosting energy and motivation

   C. Practical Uses of Essential Oils
      1. Aromatherapy and diffusing oils
      2. Topical application and massage techniques
      3. Use in household cleaning and personal care products
      4. Incorporating essential oils into a daily self-care routine

IV. Essential Oils for Specific Health Concerns
   A. Respiratory health and nasal congestion
   B. Skin conditions, acne, and aging skin
   C. Digestive issues, bloating, and indigestion
   D. Headaches, migraines, and tension
   E. Menstrual discomfort and hormonal imbalances

F. Muscular pain, joint stiffness, and inflammation

V. Essential Oils for a Healthy Home
    A. Natural cleaning alternatives using essential oils
    B. Improving indoor air quality with essential oils
    C. Creating a calming and inviting atmosphere at home
    D. Supporting a toxic-free lifestyle with essential oils

VI. Blending and Using Essential Oils
    A. Understanding the principles of blending essential oils
    B. Recipes for creating personalized blends for various purposes
    C. Different methods of application and dilution guidelines
    D. Tips for storage, shelf life, and maintaining oil quality

VII. Essential Oils Safety and Precautions
    A. Proper usage guidelines for different age groups (adults, children, infants, and
pets)
    B. Allergies, sensitivities, and potential adverse reactions
    C. Interaction with medications and other therapies
    D. Importance of sourcing high-quality and pure essential oils

VIII. Conclusion
    A. Recap the key benefits and uses of essential oils
    B. Encourage readers to explore and experiment with essential oils
    C. Emphasize the importance of consulting with a qualified healthcare professional for
specific health concerns

Introduction:

Welcome to a captivating journey through the world of essential oils, where nature's greatest gifts are distilled into tiny bottles of aromatic wonders. In this book, we will explore the immense potential and therapeutic benefits of essential oils, as well as their extraordinary role in enhancing our physical, mental, and emotional well-being.

The use of essential oils dates back centuries, with ancient civilizations harnessing the power of these fragrant essences for a myriad of purposes - from healing rituals to spiritual ceremonies and beauty regimens. Today, in a world marked by increasing stress and uncertainty, essential oils offer a natural pathway to reclaiming balance and harmony in our lives.

In this comprehensive guide, we will delve into the definition, history, and production of essential oils, immersing ourselves in their aromatic and medicinal properties. We will unravel the science behind their efficacy, exploring the intricate chemistry that imbues each oil with unique attributes and therapeutic potential.

Through meticulous research and personal experiences, this book will uncover the diverse applications of essential oils. From their capacity to reduce stress and anxiety to their ability to enhance cognitive function and support immune health, we will illuminate the many ways in which these oils can transform and uplift our daily lives.

Throughout the pages that follow, we will embark on a voyage of discovery, unveiling the ancient wisdom and modern insights that surround essential oils. We will uncover the secrets of blending oils to create customized aromatherapy blends, explore methods of optimal usage, and emphasize the importance of safety in incorporating essential oils into our routines.

Whether you are a seasoned aromatherapy enthusiast or a curious newcomer, this book seeks to empower and guide you on your aromatic pathway. It is our shared intention to foster a deeper appreciation for the marvels of nature and to awaken your senses to the extraordinary potential residing within these little bottles.

So, let us embark on this fragrant odyssey, where nature's essence intertwines with science, and where the ancient art of aromatherapy unveils its wonders. Get ready to unlock the power of essential oils and experience the transformative magic that awaits.

The Definition and History of Essential Oils

Essential oils have been used for centuries to harness the power of nature's aromatic and therapeutic benefits. Derived from various plants, essential oils are concentrated extracts that encapsulate the plant's unique characteristics. This chapter explores the definition of essential oils, their origins, and their historical significance.

Essential oils are volatile, aromatic compounds found in various parts of plants, including flowers, leaves, bark, stems, and even roots. They give each plant its distinct fragrance and are essential for the plant's survival by aiding in pollination, repelling pests, and protecting against disease.

To obtain essential oils, either steam distillation, cold pressing, or solvent extraction methods are used. Through these processes, the oil-containing glands of the plant material are ruptured, allowing the essential oil to be released and collected for further use.

The use of essential oils can be traced back thousands of years. Ancient civilizations, including the Egyptians, Greeks, and Chinese, recognized their medicinal properties and employed them in various rituals, medical practices, and cosmetics.

Egyptians, known for their advanced medical knowledge, used essential oils in embalming, religious ceremonies, and beauty rituals. They produced aromatic oils such as frankincense, myrrh, and rose oil, which were highly valued for their healing and spiritual properties.

In ancient Greece, essential oils played a pivotal role in medicine. Renowned figures like Hippocrates and Galen recognized their therapeutic value and used oils such as lavender, rosemary, and chamomile for their healing properties.

Traditional Chinese medicine also incorporated essential oils into its practices. Traditional texts, dating back to around 2000 BCE, often referred to essential oils as "chips of fragrance" and utilized them in rituals, hygiene practices, and treatments.

During the Middle Ages, essential oils became scarce in Europe due to the Byzantine Empire's downfall. The Arab world held the key to reestablishing the use of essential oils in Europe, with physicians like Avicenna contributing to their revival. Books like "De Materia Medica" by Greek physician Dioscorides further documented the medicinal potential of essential oils.

In the 19th century, with advances in botany and chemistry, essential oils began to be scientifically studied. French chemist René-Maurice Gattefossé coined the term "aromatherapy" in 1928, after experiencing the healing effects of lavender oil on his burned hand. He researched and promoted essential oils' medicinal properties, gaining widespread recognition in Europe and beyond.

The 20th century marked a boom in essential oil usage. Renowned aromatherapists, including Jean Valnet, Marguerite Maury, and Robert B. Tisserand, further expanded the understanding and application of essential oils in therapeutic practices. Their efforts led to the development of safety guidelines and the recognition of essential oils as a holistic modality.

Today, essential oils are widely used for their aromatic and therapeutic benefits. They find applications in various industries, including perfumery, cosmetics, household products, and alternative medicine. Essential oils are recognized for their ability to promote relaxation, relieve stress, enhance mood, alleviate discomfort, and support overall well-being.

Essential oils have a rich history that spans thousands of years, with civilizations recognizing and harnessing their natural medicinal properties. From ancient Egypt to modern times, essential oils have played an important role in spiritual rituals, medical practices, and even everyday life.

With advancements in science and research, their benefits and applications have become better understood, leading to increased usage and popularity. As we continue to delve into the world of essential oils, their potential seems limitless.

Whether for emotional support, physical wellness, or simply for the pleasure of experiencing their beautiful aromas, essential oils provide a connection to the past, a bridge to nature, and a pathway to holistic health.

Embracing Nature: The Growing Interest in Natural Wellness and Alternative Therapies

In recent years, there has been a significant rise in interest and engagement with natural wellness practices and alternative therapies. With the increasing awareness of the interconnectedness between our physical, mental, and emotional well-being, many individuals are seeking holistic approaches that align with nature to achieve a state of harmony and balance.

This chapter explores the reasons behind this growing interest, the benefits of natural wellness, and the various alternative therapies gaining popularity.

In a world marked by synthetic medications, high-stress levels, and modern lifestyles that often disconnect us from nature, there has been a notable shift towards embracing natural wellness practices. People are craving alternatives that nurture their well-being in gentle, sustainable ways.

One key driving factor behind this shift is the desire for a more holistic approach to health. Natural wellness practices recognize the intricate interplay between body, mind, and spirit. They aim to address the root causes of health issues rather than simply treating symptoms.

By tapping into the power of nature's resources, such as plants, essential oils, and herbal remedies, individuals can support their overall well-being on multiple levels.

Moreover, the rising interest in natural wellness can be attributed in part to increased awareness of the potential risks and side effects associated with synthetic drugs.

As people become more educated about the long-term consequences of relying solely on conventional medicine, they are turning to alternative therapies that have stood the test of time and offer a gentler, more sustainable approach to healing.

Natural wellness practices encompass a wide range of modalities and therapies, each offering its unique set of benefits. One of the key advantages is the emphasis on prevention rather than mere intervention.

Natural wellness encourages individuals to adopt a proactive approach to their health, focusing on lifestyle choices, nutrition, exercise, and stress management. By nurturing overall well-being and building a strong foundation of health, individuals are better equipped to prevent illness and maintain vitality.

Furthermore, natural wellness practices often prioritize the use of natural and organic ingredients, reducing exposure to harmful chemicals and toxins that can accumulate in our bodies over time.

This focus on purity and cleanliness extends to skincare, personal care products, and household items. Many individuals are making a conscious effort to embrace chemical-free alternatives, promoting not only their own well-being but also the health of the planet.

Additionally, natural wellness practices often incorporate alternative therapies renowned for their ability to provide relief and enhance well-being. Practices such as acupuncture, aromatherapy, massage therapy, and herbal medicine have been utilized for centuries, standing the test of time. They offer non-invasive, drug-free solutions that can help manage stress, reduce pain, improve sleep quality, and support emotional balance.

As the interest in natural wellness grows, so does the popularity of alternative therapies. People are increasingly exploring modalities that complement conventional medicine or offer standalone treatments. Acupuncture, originating in ancient China, involves the insertion of fine needles at specific points on the body to restore balance and stimulate healing. This practice is gaining recognition for its ability to alleviate pain, reduce stress, and improve overall well-being.

Aromatherapy, utilizing essential oils derived from plants, is another alternative therapy that has gained widespread popularity. The inhalation or topical application of essential oils can promote relaxation, uplift mood, aid in sleep, and address various physical and emotional concerns. Essential oils are now widely used in diffusers, skincare products, and personalized blends.

Massage therapy is yet another alternative therapy that has earned its place in mainstream wellness. Beyond providing relaxation and an escape from everyday stress, massage therapy offers benefits such as reduced muscle tension, improved circulation, and enhanced mental clarity.

The growing interest in natural wellness and alternative therapies reflects a desire for a more holistic approach to health and well-being. By embracing practices that align with nature, individuals can tap into the immense potential to nurture their mind, body, and spirit, ultimately creating a foundation for long-lasting vitality and optimal wellness.

The Essence of Nature: Understanding Essential Oils and Extraction Methods

Essential oils have gained popularity in recent years for their aromatic and therapeutic properties. Derived from various plants, these potent oils capture the essence of nature's healing powers. In this chapter, we will explore what essential oils are, how they are extracted, and the different methods used to harness their benefits.

By understanding the science and artistry behind these precious oils, we can fully appreciate their value and the ways in which they enhance our well-being.

Essential oils are concentrated, volatile compounds obtained from plant matter, such as flowers, leaves, bark, stems, and roots. These oils contain the plant's distinctive fragrance and possess numerous therapeutic properties.

As the name suggests, these oils are considered the essence or "life force" of the plant, consisting of various chemical components that interact with our bodies on a cellular level.

Essential oils can be composed of hundreds of different chemical constituents, including terpenes, phenols, alcohols, and esters, each contributing to the oil's unique characteristics and therapeutic benefits. These complex blends of constituents are carefully preserved during the extraction process.

How Are Essential Oils Extracted?

There are several methods used to extract essential oils from plants, each suited for different types of plant material and yielding different results. Here are some commonly used extraction methods:

1. Steam Distillation: This is the most common method of extracting essential oils. It involves passing steam through the plant material, causing the essential oil to evaporate and subsequently condense. The condensed vapor is then collected, and the oil is separated from the water. Steam distillation is suitable for extracting oils from flowers, leaves, and other aerial parts of plants.

2. Cold Pressing: Also known as expression, this method is primarily used for extracting essential oils from citrus fruits such as oranges, lemons, and grapefruits. It involves mechanically pressing or squeezing the peels to release the essential oils. Cold pressing ensures that the oils remain pure and free from heat-induced degradation.

3. Solvent Extraction: This method is employed when distillation or cold pressing is not feasible, such as with fragile flowers or plants that do not yield large amounts of oil. Solvent extraction involves using a solvent, usually hexane, to dissolve the essential oil from the plant material. Afterward, the solvent is evaporated, leaving behind the concentrated oil known as an absolute. Absolutes often resemble the original scent of the plant more closely but may contain trace amounts of the solvent.

4. CO2 Extraction: This method involves using carbon dioxide (CO2) in a pressurized chamber to extract essential oils. The carbon dioxide acts as both a gas and a liquid under pressure, allowing it to extract the essential oil. This method is considered highly efficient and yields high-quality oils, retaining many of the plant's delicate aromatic compounds.

5. Distillation with Water: This method, also known as hydrodistillation or water distillation, involves submerging the plant material in water and heating it. The steam produced carries the essential oil, which is then condensed and collected. This method is commonly used for plant materials that are not suitable for steam distillation alone.

Each extraction method has its advantages and considerations, and experienced distillers select the most appropriate method for each plant to obtain the desired aromatic and therapeutic qualities.

Essential oils offer a powerful connection to the natural world, harnessing the plant kingdom's extraordinary healing properties. With their unique chemical compositions and diverse extraction methods, these oils captivate our senses and promote well-being in numerous ways.

By understanding what essential oils are and how they are extracted, we gain a deep appreciation for their value and the meticulous process that allows us to experience their aromatic and therapeutic benefits.

Whether through distillation, cold pressing, or other innovative techniques, the extraction of essential oils preserves the wisdom of nature, offering us a profound connection to its healing essence.

The Science Behind Essential Oils and Their Chemical Composition

Essential oils have gained significant popularity in recent years due to their potential health benefits and therapeutic properties. However, the efficacy and safety of these potent plant extracts depend largely on their unique chemical composition and interactions with the human body. In this chapter, we will delve into the scientific aspects of essential oils, exploring their chemical constituents and understanding how they work.

Chemical Composition of Essential Oils:

Essential oils are complex mixtures of volatile compounds derived from plants. They are typically obtained through methods such as steam distillation, cold pressing, or solvent extraction. The chemical composition of essential oils can vary greatly depending on the plant species, growing conditions, harvest times, and extraction methods.

The primary constituents present in essential oils fall into several main classes, including terpenes, esters, alcohols, ketones, phenols, and aldehydes. Terpenes are the most abundant and diverse group, consisting of monoterpenes and sesquiterpenes. These hydrocarbon compounds are responsible for the distinctive fragrances and therapeutic effects associated with essential oils.

Therapeutic Potential of Essential Oils:

The therapeutic properties of essential oils can be attributed to their chemical constituents that interact with the body through different mechanisms. For instance, terpenes such as limonene and pinene possess antimicrobial properties, while menthol and linalool exhibit analgesic and anti-inflammatory effects.

Essential oils also have the ability to influence mood and emotions due to their ability to modulate neurotransmitters in the brain. For example, lavender oil contains linalool and linalyl acetate, which have been shown to promote relaxation and reduce anxiety levels. Peppermint oil, containing menthol, has been found to enhance focus and alertness when inhaled.

Interaction with the Human Body:

When applied topically, essential oils can be absorbed through the skin and enter the bloodstream. However, their fat-soluble nature enables them to penetrate cell membranes and cross the blood-brain barrier, allowing them to have systemic effects.

Once inside the body, essential oil components interact with various physiological processes. They can stimulate or inhibit enzymes, influence gene expression, and modulate receptors, thereby impacting biochemical pathways. Many essential oil compounds, such as eugenol found in clove oil, possess analgesic properties by blocking pain receptors in nerve endings.

Safety Considerations:

While essential oils are generally considered safe when used properly, it is crucial to recognize that their concentrated nature necessitates caution in their application. Some individuals may experience skin irritation or sensitivity when essential oils are directly applied. It is advisable to dilute essential oils with carrier oils before topical use and perform patch tests on a small area of skin.

Moreover, caution should be exercised when ingesting essential oils, as certain compounds may be toxic or interact adversely with medications. Always consult a qualified aromatherapist or healthcare professional for guidance on appropriate usage and dosage.

The popularity of essential oils can be attributed to their diverse chemical composition and potential therapeutic benefits. Understanding the scientific basis behind essential oils is vital to maximize their efficacy while ensuring safe usage.

By recognizing the chemical constituents and their mechanisms of action, we can harness the power of essential oils for various applications, be it for relaxation, pain relief, or mood enhancement. As with any natural product, it is crucial to exercise caution, seek professional advice, and use essential oils responsibly to fully benefit from their potential.

Exploring the Benefits of Essential Oils

Essential oils have long been cherished for their aromatic and therapeutic properties. Derived from various plant parts, these potent extracts have been used for centuries to promote physical, mental, and emotional well-being. In this chapter, we will delve into the physical benefits of essential oils, focusing on their immune-boosting properties, pain-relieving capabilities, their impact on relaxation and sleep, support for healthy digestion, and their ability to enhance skin health and beauty.

Physical Benefits:

1. Supporting the immune system and overall wellness:

Essential oils possess antimicrobial and antiviral properties that can help strengthen the immune system. Oils like tea tree, eucalyptus, and oregano are known for their potent antibacterial properties, while oils such as lemon, frankincense, and lavender have immune-enhancing effects. By diffusing these oils or applying them topically, individuals can boost their body's natural defense mechanisms, promoting overall wellness.

2. Relieving pain and inflammation:

Many essential oils have analgesic and anti-inflammatory properties, making them effective natural alternatives for pain relief and managing inflammation. For example, peppermint oil contains the compound menthol, which has been found to have a cooling effect and can help alleviate headaches and muscle pain. Similarly, lavender oil has been shown to reduce pain and inflammation in conditions such as arthritis and menstrual cramps.

3. Promoting relaxation, stress reduction, and better sleep:

One of the most well-known benefits of essential oils is their ability to promote relaxation and reduce stress. Oils like lavender, chamomile, and ylang-ylang have calming properties that can lower anxiety levels and induce a state of relaxation. By reducing stress, these oils can also improve sleep quality, making them effective aids for those struggling with insomnia or sleep disturbances.

4. Supporting healthy digestion and detoxification:

Essential oils can support healthy digestion by stimulating the release of digestive enzymes and promoting proper nutrient absorption.

Peppermint oil, for instance, has been extensively studied for its ability to relieve symptoms of irritable bowel syndrome (IBS) and indigestion. Oils such as ginger, fennel, and lemon can also aid in reducing bloating, gas, and nausea. Additionally, certain essential oils, like lemon and grapefruit, possess detoxifying properties that can support natural detoxification processes in the body.

5. Enhancing skin health and beauty:

Essential oils have been widely used in skincare for their ability to improve the health, appearance, and texture of the skin. Tea tree oil, known for its antibacterial and antifungal properties, can help combat acne and blemishes.

Similarly, oils such as rosehip, geranium, and frankincense aid in reducing the signs of aging, promoting a youthful complexion, and improving overall skin health. Their antioxidant properties help protect the skin from environmental damage and support collagen production.

From supporting the immune system and relieving pain to promoting relaxation, aiding digestion, and enhancing skin health, essential oils offer a wide array of physical benefits. Through their unique chemical composition and interactions with the body, these aromatic compounds have demonstrated therapeutic potential. However, it is important to note that essential oils should be used responsibly and with proper guidance.

Consultation with a qualified aromatherapist or healthcare professional is recommended to determine the most suitable oils and methods of application for individual needs. By incorporating essential oils into a well-balanced lifestyle, individuals can harness their natural properties to support physical well-being and unlock a world of benefits.

Exploring the Emotional and Mental Benefits of Essential Oils

Essential oils have long been valued for their soothing and uplifting aromatic properties. Not only do these natural extracts offer physical benefits, but they also possess powerful emotional and mental advantages. In this chapter we will delve into the emotional and mental benefits of essential oils, focusing on their ability to uplift mood, reduce anxiety and stress, enhance cognitive function, support emotional balance, and boost energy and motivation.

1. Uplifting mood and reducing anxiety, stress, and depression:
Essential oils have the remarkable ability to influence emotions and uplift mood. Oils like bergamot, citrus, and clary sage are known for their uplifting properties and can help combat feelings of anxiety, stress, and depression. The inhalation of these oils through diffusers or personal inhalers stimulates the limbic system, promoting the release of neurotransmitters like serotonin and dopamine, which are responsible for regulating mood and emotions.

2. Enhancing focus, concentration, and mental clarity:

Certain essential oils have been found to improve focus, concentration, and mental clarity. Rosemary oil, for example, has been shown to enhance cognitive performance and memory. Peppermint oil can boost alertness and stimulate mental clarity, making it useful for tasks that require sustained attention. These oils can be diffused, used in a personal inhaler, or diluted and applied topically for optimal concentration and focus during work or studying.

3. Supporting emotional balance and well-being:

Essential oils can play a significant role in supporting emotional balance and overall well-being. Oils such as lavender, roman chamomile, and ylang-ylang possess calming properties that help reduce feelings of irritability, restlessness, and emotional tension. By promoting relaxation and soothing the nervous system, these oils contribute to emotional stability and enhanced well-being.

4. Boosting energy and motivation:

Feeling tired or lacking energy can be a common occurrence in today's fast-paced world. Thankfully, essential oils can offer a natural solution. Oils like citrus (such as lemon and grapefruit) and peppermint are known for their invigorating and uplifting properties. These oils can be diffused or applied topically to provide an energizing boost and enhance motivation, making them beneficial for combating fatigue and maintaining focus throughout the day.

Essential oils go beyond their pleasant aroma and offer a myriad of emotional and mental benefits. From uplifting mood and reducing anxiety, stress, and depression to enhancing focus, concentration, and mental clarity, these natural extracts have the potential to positively impact our emotional and mental well-being.

Through their influence on the limbic system and neurotransmitter regulation, essential oils can support emotional balance and promote a sense of tranquility. Additionally, their invigorating properties can boost energy and motivation, making them valuable aids in combating fatigue and maintaining mental alertness.

To harness the full potential of essential oils, it is recommended to consult with a qualified aromatherapist or healthcare professional for guidance on appropriate oils, methods of application, and an individualized approach for emotional and mental support. Incorporating essential oils into a balanced lifestyle can contribute to a greater sense of well-being and enhanced emotional and mental health.

Practical Uses of Essential Oils

Essential oils are versatile and potent natural extracts that offer a wide range of benefits. From promoting relaxation to supporting physical and emotional well-being, these aromatic compounds have numerous practical applications. In this chapter, we will explore some of the practical uses of essential oils, including aromatherapy and diffusing oils, topical application and massage techniques, utilizing them in household cleaning and personal care products, and incorporating them into a daily self-care routine.

1. Aromatherapy and diffusing oils:

Perhaps the most well-known use of essential oils is through aromatherapy and diffusing. By using an essential oil diffuser, individuals can disperse the aroma of their chosen oil throughout a room, creating a pleasant and therapeutic atmosphere. This method allows for inhalation of the aromatic compounds, which can influence mood, emotions, and overall well-being. Whether one seeks relaxation, upliftment, or focus, diffusing essential oils can provide a desired effect.

2. Topical application and massage techniques:

Topical application of essential oils can yield numerous benefits. When properly diluted with carrier oils, such as coconut or jojoba oil, essential oils can be safely applied to the skin. Massage techniques involving essential oils can help promote relaxation, relieve muscle tension, and support improved circulation. Applying oils to specific areas, such as temples or pulse points, can target specific concerns, such as headaches or stress.

3. Use in household cleaning and personal care products:

Essential oils are not limited to therapeutic applications; they can also be utilized in practical ways around the house. Many essential oils possess antimicrobial and antiseptic properties, making them valuable additions to natural cleaning solutions.

Tea tree oil, for example, can be added to homemade counter sprays or laundry detergent to enhance their disinfecting properties. Furthermore, essential oils can be incorporated into personal care products like soaps, shampoos, and lotions, providing a natural and aromatic alternative to chemical-laden products.

4. Incorporating essential oils into a daily self-care routine:

Incorporating essential oils into a daily self-care routine can be a wonderful way to support overall well-being. Essential oils can be added to bathwater for a relaxing and therapeutic soak. Adding a few drops of lavender oil to a pillow or bedding can promote a restful night's sleep.

Using essential oils in a facial steam or as part of a skincare routine can offer rejuvenating properties for the skin. By incorporating essential oils into daily rituals, individuals can experience the numerous benefits they have to offer.

Essential oils have practical uses in various aspects of life, encompassing aromatherapy, topical application, household cleaning, and personal care. Whether diffusing oils for therapeutic purposes, incorporating them into massages or skincare routines, or utilizing their antimicrobial properties in cleaning solutions, essential oils offer practical and natural solutions for various needs.

As with any natural product, it is important to use essential oils responsibly and seek guidance from qualified professionals regarding appropriate usage and dilution ratios. By incorporating essential oils into daily routines, individuals can enhance their well-being and experience the numerous practical benefits these natural extracts have to offer.

Essential oils have long been used for their various health benefits and can be particularly effective in addressing specific health concerns. When it comes to respiratory health and nasal congestion, oils such as eucalyptus, peppermint, and tea tree can help clear airways and alleviate symptoms.

For those struggling with skin conditions, acne, or signs of aging, lavender, frankincense, and geranium are popular choices known for their soothing and rejuvenating properties.

Digestive issues, bloating, and indigestion can be eased with oils like ginger, peppermint, and fennel that can support digestion and provide relief. Headaches, migraines, and tension can be effectively managed with oils such as lavender, peppermint, and rosemary, which possess calming and pain-relieving properties.

Menstrual discomfort and hormonal imbalances can be addressed through the use of oils like clary sage, lavender, and chamomile, renowned for their balancing and soothing effects.

Finally, muscular pain, joint stiffness, and inflammation can be relieved with oils such as peppermint, marjoram, and helichrysum that have anti-inflammatory and analgesic properties, promoting relaxation and pain relief.

Essential oils can be used effectively to address respiratory health and nasal congestion by employing various methods of application. One popular method is inhalation, where a few drops of the essential oil are added to a diffuser or a bowl of hot water, allowing the aromatic molecules to disperse into the air and be inhaled.

This can help clear the airways, reduce congestion, and promote easier breathing. Another option is to apply the essential oil topically, by diluting a few drops in a carrier oil like coconut or jojoba oil, and massaging it onto the chest, neck, and back. This allows the oil to be absorbed through the skin and provide localized relief. Lastly, some essential oils like eucalyptus and peppermint can also be added to a warm bath, creating a soothing steam that can help open up congested airways.

Using essential oils for skin conditions, acne, and aging skin can be a transformative experience, leaving you with a rejuvenated and radiant complexion. These potent, natural extracts have long been cherished for their therapeutic properties, harnessing the power of nature to address various skin concerns. For those struggling with acne, essential oils like tea tree oil or lavender can work wonders by calming inflammation, reducing redness, and fighting off pesky breakouts.

When it comes to addressing aging skin, essential oils such as rosehip oil or frankincense oil can work miracles, promoting collagen production, reducing the appearance of fine lines and wrinkles, and restoring a youthful glow. The fragrant and uplifting nature of these oils not only leaves your skin feeling nourished, but also uplifts your spirits, instilling a sense of optimism and confidence in your skincare routine. So, embark on this aromatic journey and embrace the transformative power of essential oils for your skin!

Using essential oils for bloating, digestive issues, and indigestion can provide you with natural relief and a renewed sense of vitality. These aromatic extracts have been cherished for centuries for their ability to soothe and support the digestive system, offering a gentle and holistic approach to combating these common discomforts.

When it comes to bloating, essential oils like peppermint or ginger can work wonders by relaxing the muscles in the gastrointestinal tract, reducing inflammation, and promoting healthy digestion. Their invigorating and refreshing scent not only uplifts your spirits but also helps to alleviate the discomfort often associated with bloating.

For those struggling with digestive issues, essential oils such as fennel or chamomile can provide much-needed relief by calming the stomach, reducing spasms, and easing indigestion. The soothing properties of these oils can help restore balance to your digestive system, allowing you to enjoy your meals without any discomfort.

Whether you're dealing with occasional bouts of indigestion or chronic digestive issues, essential oils offer a natural and optimistic solution, empowering you to take control of your digestive health. So, embrace the power of these uplifting and aromatic extracts, and enjoy a renewed sense of wellness and optimism for your digestive system.

Essential oils can be a natural and soothing remedy for migraines and tension headaches, offering relief and promoting a sense of calm and relaxation. These powerful plant extracts have been utilized for centuries for their therapeutic properties, and when used correctly, they can provide effective relief from these debilitating conditions.

One popular essential oil for migraines is lavender oil, known for its calming and stress-relieving properties. Applying a few drops to your temples or inhaling the aroma can help ease the intensity of migraines and promote relaxation.

Peppermint oil is another go-to option, as it has a cooling effect and can help alleviate tension and reduce pain. Simply dilute a few drops of peppermint oil with a carrier oil, and gently massage onto the temples, forehead, or neck. Eucalyptus oil is also known for its analgesic and anti-inflammatory properties, offering relief from headaches caused by sinus congestion or tension.

By adding a few drops to a diffuser or inhaling the steam from a warm bowl of water infused with the oil, you can experience its therapeutic benefits. Ultimately, the use of essential oils for migraines and tension headaches provides a holistic and optimistic approach to managing these conditions, promoting relaxation, and a renewed sense of well-being.

Using essential oils for menstrual discomfort and hormonal imbalances can be a gentle and natural way to find relief and support your overall well-being. These powerful plant extracts have been used for centuries to help balance hormones, reduce inflammation, and ease the discomfort associated with menstruation.

One of the most popular essential oils for menstrual discomfort is clary sage, known for its calming and balancing properties. By applying a few drops of clary sage diluted in a carrier oil, such as coconut or jojoba oil, directly to your lower abdomen, you can help reduce cramps and provide a soothing sensation.

Lavender essential oil is another great choice for its calming effects and ability to alleviate tension and stress. Diffusing lavender oil during your menstrual cycle or adding a few drops to a warm bath can promote relaxation and balance. Lastly, geranium essential oil is known for its hormone-regulating properties.

By applying a few drops on your wrists or adding it to a massage oil, you can help regulate your menstrual cycle and reduce hormonal imbalances. Remember, every woman is unique, so it's essential to listen to your body and find the combinations that work best for you. Just be sure to dilute essential oils properly and perform a patch test before applying them to your skin. With patience and experimentation, essential oils can become a valuable tool in your wellness routine, supporting you through the ups and downs of your menstrual cycle.

If you're struggling with muscular pain, joint stiffness, or inflammation, incorporating the use of essential oils into your daily routine may be just the thing you need to find relief and support your overall well-being. Essential oils have long been praised for their therapeutic properties, and many of them possess powerful anti-inflammatory and analgesic effects that can help ease discomfort in the muscles and joints.

Oils such as lavender, peppermint, and eucalyptus can be particularly beneficial in reducing inflammation, promoting relaxation, and improving circulation. When combined with proper rest, gentle stretching, and a healthy lifestyle, the regular use of essential oils can help you overcome these challenges and regain your mobility and comfort.

Experiment with different blends and methods of application, such as diluting a few drops of essential oil in a carrier oil and massaging it onto the affected area, or adding a few drops to a warm bath to soak in. Give your body the nurturing care it deserves and embrace the healing power of essential oils.

Creating a Healthy Home environment involves being mindful of indoor air quality, and one effective way to purify and improve the air we breathe is by incorporating essential oils. These natural plant extracts not only emit delightful scents but also possess fantastic air-cleansing properties. For instance, eucalyptus oil is renowned for its ability to ward off airborne bacteria and viruses, making it an excellent choice for reducing the risk of respiratory ailments.

Additionally, tea tree oil can combat mold and mildew, eliminating potential allergens and irritants from the air. Citrus-based oils, such as lemon or orange, serve as natural air fresheners, purifying the atmosphere while uplifting our spirits with their vibrant aromas. By diffusing these essential oils regularly, we can transform our homes into havens of cleanliness and vitality, ensuring that the air we breathe is not only pure but also invigorating.

Creating a Calming and Inviting Atmosphere at Home with Essential Oils

In the midst of today's hectic and stressful lifestyles, it's crucial to create a calming and inviting atmosphere in our homes—a sanctuary where we can unwind, rejuvenate, and find inner peace. One effective way to achieve this is by using essential oils. Derived from plants, these natural extracts possess aromatic properties that can promote relaxation, reduce anxiety, and uplift our mood. In this chapter, we'll explore the best essential oils for creating a tranquil atmosphere, discuss various methods of diffusion, and provide tips on incorporating essential oils into your daily routine to energize and harmonize your home.

Choosing the Right Essential Oils:

When it comes to creating a calming atmosphere, several essential oils stand out for their soothing scents and therapeutic benefits. Lavender oil, renowned for its calming and sleep-inducing properties, is perfect for bedrooms and relaxation spaces. The invigorating aroma of citrus oils, such as orange and bergamot, can breathe life into living areas, while geranium oil creates a serene atmosphere and promotes emotional balance. Essential oils like ylang-ylang and clary sage blend harmoniously to cultivate a peaceful ambiance.

Diffusion Techniques:

Once you've selected your essential oils, it's important to know how to effectively disperse their aromatic molecules into the air. Diffusers, available in various types such as ultrasonic, nebulizer, or reed diffusers, are a popular choice. Ultrasonic diffusers use electronic frequencies to emit a fine mist of essential oil-infused water, while nebulizers break down the oil for efficient diffusion. Reed diffusers use reeds to draw oil up and disperse the scent naturally.

Another easy and cost-effective diffusion method is steam inhalation. Simply add a few drops of your chosen oil to a bowl of hot water and inhale the fragrant steam. Oil burners and candle warmers provide simultaneous fragrance and visual appeal, while topical application, such as massage oils or bath products, allows for a more intimate experience with essential oils.

Incorporating Essential Oils Into Your Daily Routine:

Creating a calming and inviting home atmosphere extends beyond diffusion techniques. Here are some tips for effectively incorporating essential oils into your daily routine to promote relaxation and well-being:

1. Bedtime Rituals: Enhance your sleep routine by adding a drop of lavender oil onto your pillow or using a linen spray infused with soothing oils to create a serene sleep environment.

2. Meditation and Yoga: Diffuse grounding oils like frankincense, sandalwood, or patchouli during your meditation or yoga sessions to create a peaceful ambiance and deepen your practice.

3. Bathroom Bliss: Transform your bathroom into a serene spa-like retreat by adding a few drops of essential oils to your bathwater or shower gel. Eucalyptus and peppermint oils are excellent choices for promoting invigorating and uplifting experiences.

4. Scented Linens and Fabrics: Create a welcoming atmosphere by adding a few drops of your favorite essential oil onto fabric softener or dryer sheets. This will infuse your linens, curtains, and upholstery with a gentle and refreshing fragrance.

5. Desk Diffusion: Combat stress and boost focus during work or study sessions by diffusing essential oils like rosemary, lemon, or peppermint near your desk. These scents can promote mental clarity and enhance productivity.

6. Seasonal Blends: Tailor your essential oil blends to create a cozy atmosphere that suits each season. For instance, cloves and cinnamon evoke warmth during winter, while floral notes like jasmine and rose embody spring's renewal.

Essential oils offer a natural and effective way to transform your home into a haven of tranquility and comfort. By carefully choosing the right oils, utilizing various diffusion techniques, and incorporating them into your everyday routines, you can create an inviting atmosphere that promotes relaxation, reduces anxiety, and enhances overall well-being. Embrace the power of essential oils, and let their aromatic molecules carry you to a world of serenity within the walls of your home.

Embrace a Toxic-Free Lifestyle with Essential Oils

Living a toxic-free lifestyle has become increasingly vital in our modern world. The harmful chemicals found in everyday products can negatively impact our health and the environment. Thankfully, essential oils offer a natural alternative that supports a toxic-free lifestyle.

These plant-derived extracts contain potent compounds that provide a range of benefits, from cleaning and disinfecting to promoting overall well-being. In this chapter, we'll explore the various ways essential oils can help you eliminate toxins from your daily life and create a healthier, more sustainable environment for you and your loved ones.

Cleaning and Disinfecting:

One of the most significant contributors to toxic exposure is conventional cleaning products. Many contain harsh chemicals such as bleach, ammonia, and synthetic fragrances, which can cause respiratory issues and irritate the skin. Essential oils, however, offer powerful cleaning properties without the harmful side effects.

Tea tree oil, known for its antimicrobial properties, can be used to clean surfaces, floors, and even laundry. Lemon oil is a natural grease cutter and can be added to DIY cleaning solutions for a fresh and effective eco-friendly cleaner. Additionally, eucalyptus, lavender, or peppermint oils can be diffused while cleaning to purify the air and provide a refreshing scent without artificial fragrances.

Personal Care and Beauty Products:

Many personal care and beauty products contain toxic chemicals that can disrupt our hormonal balance and adversely affect our well-being. Essential oils provide a natural alternative, allowing us to create our own non-toxic products or choose from a growing range of essential oil-infused options available in the market. For instance, tea tree oil can be added to shampoo to address dandruff and promote scalp health, while lavender oil can soothe skin irritations and support a healthy complexion.

DIY recipes for natural deodorants, toothpaste, and facial cleansers are readily available, offering a safer and more sustainable approach to personal care.

Aromatherapy and Emotional Well-being:

Emotional well-being is an essential aspect of a toxic-free lifestyle. Stress, anxiety, and mental fatigue take a toll on our overall health. Essential oils have been used for centuries in aromatherapy to support emotional balance and uplift the spirit. Oils such as lavender, chamomile, and bergamot have calming properties that assist in reducing stress and promoting relaxation.

Energizing oils like peppermint and citrus oils can provide a boost of positivity and focus throughout the day. By incorporating essential oils into our self-care routines, such as diffusing them, creating personalized essential oil blends, or using them in relaxing baths, we can nurture our mental and emotional well-being naturally.

Embracing a toxic-free lifestyle with essential oils benefits both our health and the environment. By replacing conventional cleaning products with essential oil-based alternatives, we eliminate exposure to harmful chemicals while maintaining a clean and fresh home. Similarly, choosing non-toxic personal care and beauty products infused with essential oils helps us avoid unnecessary chemical exposure and supports healthier skin and hair.

Moreover, incorporating essential oils into our daily routines through aromatherapy promotes emotional well-being and reduces stress levels. By harnessing the power of essential oils, we can create a healthier, safer, and more sustainable lifestyle that is free from toxins.

Discovering the Art of Blending and Using Essential Oils: The Principles, Recipes, Application Methods, and Storage Tips

Essential oils have gained immense popularity in recent years for their natural therapeutic benefits and versatility. Understanding the art of blending and using essential oils is essential to harness their full potential.

This comprehensive guide will delve into the principles of blending, share recipes for personalized blends, explore various methods of application and dilution guidelines, and provide tips for proper storage and maintaining oil quality. Whether you're a seasoned aromatherapist or a beginner, this chapter aims to deepen your knowledge and empower you to create custom, effective essential oil blends for various purposes.

Part 1: Principles of Blending Essential Oils:

1. Importance of Synergy: Essential oils interact with each other, creating a synergistic effect that enhances their individual properties. Understanding the characteristics, therapeutic properties, and fragrance notes of each oil helps in creating balanced blends

2. Top, Middle, and Base Notes: Essential oils are classified into top, middle, and base notes based on their evaporation rates and intensity. Blending oils from each category creates a well-rounded aroma that unfolds over time.

3. Scent Families: Essential oils belong to specific scent families, such as floral, citrus, woody, or herbal. Mixing oils from the same family often leads to pleasing combinations, but experimenting with different scent families can provide unique and exciting results.

4. Dilution Ratios: An understanding of dilution ratios ensures safe and effective use of essential oils. Different applications require varying dilution strengths to achieve desired results while avoiding skin irritation or sensitization.

Part 2: Recipes for Creating Personalized Blends:

1. Relaxing and Calming Blend for Stress Relief: Combining lavender, chamomile, and bergamot essential oils creates a soothing blend perfect for relaxation, reducing anxiety, and promoting restful sleep.

2. Energizing Blend for Mental Focus: Utilize invigorating oils like peppermint, rosemary, and lemon for a stimulating blend that can enhance concentration and mental clarity.

3. Respiratory Support Blend: Eucalyptus, tea tree, and thyme essential oils blended together can help clear congestion, support the respiratory system, and alleviate symptoms of cold or flu.

4. Mood-Boosting Blend: Create a cheerful and uplifting blend by combining citrus oils like orange, grapefruit, and lemon, which are known for their ability to uplift the mood and boost positivity.

5. Immune Support Blend: A blend of clove, cinnamon, and orange essential oils can help strengthen the immune system and provide natural antiviral and antibacterial properties.

Part 3: Methods of Application and Dilution Guidelines:

1. Inhalation: Direct inhalation, steam inhalation, and using diffusers are effective methods for harnessing the aromatic benefits of essential oils.

2. Topical Application: Diluting essential oils in carrier oils, such as coconut, jojoba, or almond oil, is crucial to avoid sensitization or irritation. Dilution ratios vary depending on the age, sensitivity, and intended use.

3. Baths and Massage: Adding essential oils to bathwater or using them in massage oils enhances relaxation, promotes muscle relief, and supports overall well-being.

4. Compresses and Sprays: Using essential oils in compresses or creating homemade sprays allows for targeted application on specific areas of the body or in the environment.

Part 4: Tips for Storage, Shelf Life, and Maintaining Oil Quality:

1. Proper Storage: Essential oils should be stored in dark glass bottles, away from direct sunlight, heat, and moisture, to maintain their potency.

2. Shelf Life: Essential oils generally have a shelf life of 1-3 years. However, citrus oils tend to have a shorter shelf life. Regularly assessing the aroma and appearance of oils is crucial to ensure their quality.

3. Cold Pressed vs. Steam Distilled: Understanding the extraction methods used for each oil helps in determining their shelf life and potential for oxidation.

4. Quality Control: It is important to source high-quality, pure essential oils from reputable manufacturers or suppliers to ensure their therapeutic benefits and avoid contaminants or dilution.

Blending and using essential oils is an art that combines knowledge, creativity, and intuition. By understanding the principles of blending, experimenting with various recipes, exploring different application methods, and following proper storage and maintenance guidelines, individuals can harness the full potential of essential oils. Whether for relaxation, enhancing focus, supporting the immune system, or simply creating a pleasing aroma, personalized essential oil blends offer limitless possibilities for well-being and enjoyment.

With this comprehensive guide, you are equipped with the knowledge and tools to embark on a journey of self-discovery and optimal health through the world of essential oils.

Harnessing the Power of Essential Oils: A Recap of Key Benefits and Uses

Essential oils have been used for centuries across various cultures and traditions for their healing and therapeutic properties. Their natural and aromatic nature offers numerous health benefits and versatile uses. Throughout this article, we've explored the many advantages of essential oils, discussed their diverse applications, and highlighted the importance of consulting qualified healthcare professionals for personalized guidance.

Recap of Key Benefits:

Essential oils possess a wide range of benefits that positively impact both the physical and mental well-being of individuals. These benefits include:

1. Aromatherapy and Emotional Well-being:

The power of essential oils in aromatherapy cannot be underestimated. Different scents can evoke various emotions, uplift moods, and promote relaxation. Oils such as lavender, chamomile, and bergamot have been proven to alleviate stress, reduce anxiety, and improve sleep quality.

2. Natural First Aid:

Essential oils act as potent natural antiseptics, antimicrobials, and anti-inflammatories, providing effective relief for minor wounds, cuts, and insect bites. Tea tree oil and lavender oil are known for their remarkable healing properties and can help soothe the skin and promote faster recovery.

3. Respiratory and Immune System Support:

Many essential oils possess volatile compounds that can help ease respiratory issues, stimulate immune responses, and alleviate symptoms related to the common cold, cough, sinus infections, and allergies. Eucalyptus, peppermint, and lemon oils are particularly beneficial for respiratory health.

4. Pain Relief and Muscle Relaxation:

Essential oils like peppermint, ginger, and lavender can aid in reducing pain and muscle tension when applied topically. Their analgesic and anti-inflammatory properties provide a natural alternative for managing headaches, menstrual cramps, joint pain, and muscle soreness.

5. Skin and Hair Care:

Utilizing essential oils in skincare routines can help address various dermatological concerns. Tea tree oil, chamomile oil, and rosehip oil possess anti-inflammatory and antioxidant properties that can help treat acne, soothe irritation, and promote healthy skin rejuvenation. Additionally, oils like rosemary and cedarwood can be beneficial in promoting hair growth and managing dandruff.

Recap of Key Uses:

The versatility of essential oils allows for numerous applications, enhancing various aspects of our lives. Some of the prominent uses of essential oils include:

1. Diffusion:

Dispersing essential oils in the air via diffusers or nebulizers allows inhalation of therapeutic aromas, promoting relaxation, concentration, and emotional balance.

2. Massage:

Blending essential oils with carrier oils for massage therapy enhances relaxation, reduces muscle tension, and promotes overall well-being.

3. Bathing:

Add a few drops of essential oil to your bathwater for a soothing and aromatic bath experience. This helps unwind, promotes relaxation, and facilitates better sleep.

4. Inhalation:

Inhaling essential oils either directly from a bottle or a handkerchief can help open up air passageways, alleviate congestion, and offer quick relief during respiratory distress.

Warning and Precautions:

While essential oils provide numerous benefits, it is crucial to consult with a qualified healthcare professional, particularly for any individual concerns. Essential oils can interact with certain medications or medical conditions, and professional guidance ensures safe and effective usage. Pregnant women, young children, and those with chronic illnesses should exercise caution and consult medical experts before incorporating essential oils into their routines.

Encourage Exploration and Experimentation:

Understanding the benefits and uses of essential oils is just the beginning of harnessing their potential. Encourage readers to explore and experiment with different oils, blends, and methods of application. Keep in mind that everyone's experience may vary, and finding the most suitable oils for individual needs often requires trial and error.

The world of essential oils offers a vast array of benefits and uses that have been celebrated for centuries. From promoting emotional balance to providing natural first aid, essential oils have the potential to revolutionize our well-being routines.

However, it is crucial to remember that while essential oils are generally safe, personalized guidance from qualified healthcare professionals is paramount when dealing with specific health concerns. Through responsible exploration and expert advice, essential oils can become an integral part of a holistic approach to improve overall health and quality of life.

Essential Oils Safety and Precautions: Guidelines for Proper Usage and Considerations

While essential oils offer numerous therapeutic benefits, it is crucial to understand the importance of safety and precautions. This comprehensive guide explores essential oil safety guidelines for different age groups, including adults, children, infants, and pets.

We will also discuss allergies, sensitivities, and potential adverse reactions, the interaction of essential oils with medications and other therapies, and the significance of sourcing high-quality and pure essential oils. By following these guidelines and being informed, you can safely and effectively harness the power of essential oils for your well-being and that of your loved ones.

Part 1: Essential Oil Safety for Different Age Groups:

1. Adults: Guidelines for proper dilution ratios, recommended oils, and application methods for adults, including considerations for pregnant and breastfeeding individuals.

2. Children: Essential oil safety precautions for children, including age-specific dilution ratios, suitable oils, and safe application methods. Attention to age, size, and overall health should be taken into account.

3. Infants: Special considerations for essential oil use with infants, including proper dilution ratios, safe oils, and recommended application methods. Extra caution is required due to their sensitive skin and developing systems.

4. Pets: Safety precautions when using essential oils around pets, including oils to avoid and proper methods of diffusion. Some essential oils can be harmful or toxic to certain animals.

Part 2: Allergies, Sensitivities, and Potential Adverse Reactions:

1. Allergic Reactions: Understanding the difference between allergies and sensitivities and recognizing common symptoms of an allergic reaction to essential oils. Patch testing and gradual introduction of oils are vital precautions.

2. Skin Sensitization: Essential oils can cause skin sensitization or irritation if used improperly or in excessive amounts. Tips for performing a patch test, recognizing signs of sensitization, and prevention strategies.

3. Photosensitivity: Certain essential oils, particularly citrus oils, can cause photosensitivity, leading to increased sunburn risk or skin discoloration. Precautions to minimize photosensitivity and safe sun exposure practices.

4. Inhalation Sensitivities: Awareness of potential respiratory sensitivities to essential oil inhalation and recognizing symptoms of respiratory distress. Proper ventilation and avoiding prolonged exposure to strong aromatic oils are key.

Part 3: Interaction with Medications and Other Therapies:

1. Medication Interactions: Understanding possible interactions between essential oils and prescription medications or over-the-counter drugs. Precautions for individuals on medication to avoid adverse effects or reduced efficacy.

2. Complementary Therapies: Coordinating the use of essential oils with other complementary therapies, such as homeopathy or acupuncture. Understanding potential synergistic effects or conflicts is crucial for optimal results.

3. Medical Conditions: Consultation with a healthcare professional is essential when using essential oils for individuals with specific medical conditions, such as asthma, epilepsy, or hormonal imbalances.

4. Aromatherapy and Massage Therapy: Guidelines for practicing safe aromatherapy or receiving essential oil-infused massages from trained and qualified professionals.

Part 4: Importance of Sourcing High-Quality and Pure Essential Oils:

1. Label Reading: Understanding the information on essential oil labels, including botanical names, country of origin, and testing certification. Look for reputable suppliers who conduct third-party testing.

2. Adulteration and Contamination: Risks associated with adulterated and contaminated essential oils, including reduced therapeutic benefits and potential health hazards. The importance of sourcing from reputable suppliers who prioritize quality and purity.

3. Organic and Ethical Sourcing: Choosing organic essential oils ensures you avoid harmful pesticides and support sustainable farming practices. Ethical sourcing ensures respect for the environment and fair labor practices.

4. Essential Oil Storage: Proper storage techniques to maintain oil quality, including keeping oils in dark glass bottles, away from direct sunlight, heat, and moisture.

Essential oils can provide remarkable benefits when used safely and responsibly. By adhering to proper usage guidelines for different age groups, understanding potential allergies and sensitivities, recognizing interactions with medications and other therapies, and sourcing high-quality and pure essential oils, you can enjoy the therapeutic advantages of these natural extracts.

Remember to consult health professionals when needed and approach essential oil use with caution and informed decision-making. With knowledge and thoughtful choices, you can enhance your well-being while prioritizing safety and precautionary measures.